Magnet Therapy

New Dawn

NEW DAWN
a division of Sterling Publishers (P) Ltd.
A-59, Okhla Industrial Area, New Delhi-110020
Ph.: 26387070, 26386209 Fax: 91-11-26383788
E-mail: ghai@nde.vsnl.net.in
Internet: http://www.sterlingpublishers.com

Magnet Therapy

ISBN 81 207 2635 9

Published by Sterling Publishers Pvt. Ltd., New Delhi-110020.
Lasertypeset by Vikas Compographics, New Delhi-110020.
Printed at Sai Early Learners Pvt. Ltd., New Delhi-110020.

Contents

Preface

It is believed that the human body possesses vital energy. This energy gives life to the whole system. It is derived from the mother's womb initially, then from the food we eat and drink, the air we breathe, and above all from the biggest source of energy, the sun.

If the energy levels in the human body are lowered, it leads to sickness.

Magnets are a source of natural energy. Magnet Therapy, through the use of different types of magnets helps maintain balanced energy levels and also increases the curative power of an individual.

Introduction

Magnetism is a type of energy present in the universe. It is the force of attraction present between the two opposite poles, whether it is electrical charges like negative and positive poles or the geographical poles — North Pole and South Pole. Opposite poles attract each other while similar poles repel each other.

Every substance or rather every particle in the universe possesses some amount of magnetic energy. Internally, this force of attraction is due to the atomic structure of each substance, where the number of electrons determine the amount of magnetic energy in that substance.

In an atom, the nucleus has protons and neutrons which are positively charged, thus making the nucleus also positively charged. Outside the nucleus, the electrons are arranged in different orbits that carry the negative charge. It is the force of attraction between the electrons and the nucleus that gives magnetism to the atom. So the atom is not free of electrical charges also. The force of attraction creates a magnetic field between the two poles while the actual movement of electrons causes the electrical energy flow.

A similar configuration is seen in the universe also. The sun is considered as the largest magnetic body. It is believed that all planetary bodies have originated from the sun.

The fragmented bodies got separated from the sun, but could not break themselves from its magnetic field. This made them revolve around the sun. It is the magnetic force of attraction of the sun that makes the earth and other planets revolve round the sun in a fixed orbit. The sun becomes the nucleus and the planets revolve around it in a fixed orbit, due to the force of attraction between the two. Hence, it is the magnetic energy that holds the various planets in their orbits and makes them revolve around the sun. The earth, being one of the planets, also has a magnetism of its own with its poles synchronising with the geographical poles.

All the planets are attracted towards the sun due its magnetic energy or force, but at the same time they also have magnetic energy of their own. The earth also has magnetic energy of its own, with a magnetic field extending up to a distance of 1,05,600 kilometres around it. It is believed that such strong magnetism has been acquired by the earth due to the constant rotation of the earth on its axis and revolution around the sun. This makes the earth a single strong magnet with two poles — the North Pole and the South Pole. This also exerts a direct and deep penetrating effect on all the objects on the earth — living and nonliving. As the planets are magnetised by the sun, the objects on the earth are also magnetised by the earth's magnetism. It is because of this magnetic force of the earth that all objects stick to the earth, and do not fly off into the atmosphere. Hence, every cell or rather every atom is magnetised.

Every atom is affected by the earth's magnetic force and has magnetic energy of its own. Every atom becomes an individual magnet.

If we see the atomic structure of any atom, we find it is very similar to the arrangement of the heavenly bodies in the universe. We find as the sun is in the center and attracts the planets towards it, or maintains the orbital distance of their revolution, so does an atom. The atom has a nucleus at the center and is positively charged, while the electrons revolve round it in their own fixed orbits, carrying opposite negative charge. This makes each atom also an independent magnet. This small magnet then has its own magnetic field and own force of attraction that binds it to the surrounding atoms to form different molecules and so on.

The earth as a huge independent magnet, exerts its influence on all living cells also, and has a great effect on the health and vitality of all living beings. It is given in our *Vedas* that —

- We should walk barefooted on green grass. It helps us to wash away fatigue and it restores health by providing us magnetic energy and thus compensating for the energy lost during the day.
- In Naturopathy, many diseases of the skin, arthritis, polio, paralysis, stomach ailments, etc, are treated by mud or sand. Mud packs are applied to the affected area of the body continuously for some days and the patient is asked to lie in the sun. It is not the mud that cures but the earth's magnetic energy that is passed on to the ailing body which cures the ailment. All diseases are caused because of lack of energy in an organ and when that energy is replenished by the earth's magnetic energy, the organ begins to restore its healthy condition.
- The Hindus have a religious custom to take down the body of a dying person from the cot and lay it on the floor, the head facing the north and the feet towards the south direction. It is

believed that the spontaneous flow of earth's magnetic energy through the body reduces the death pangs and lessens the agony of separating the vital force from the physical body.

- The *Vaastu* science is also based on this phenomenon. We have to live in harmony with nature and not against it. Therefore, it is important to follow the laws of nature. The house should be built according to the magnetic field at a given spot on the earth and the direction of the solar energy to live a healthy life. For example, our beds should be so directed that when we lie down, our head should be in the north direction and the feet should face the south. Then we can get a sound sleep and wake up in the morning feeling fresh. This is done, so that there is an easy flow of magnetic energy through our body when we are in line with the earth's magnetic field.

Certain substances exhibit the actual flow or movements of electrons in the atoms. These are called magnets. They are capable of creating an actual magnetic field whereby all objects in the domain of this field are attracted towards it.

What Are Magnets?

A magnet, so called, got its name from a place in Greece called Magnesia. This mineral was mined in this province as Magnetite. Hence, it derived its name 'magnet'. The Greeks called it *Magnetic*, or *Magnetos*. The English called it *Lodestone* because of its property of always pointing towards the North and thus indicating the direction. The French named it *Ament* or *Loving Stone* while the Indians called it *Chumbak*, the kissing stone. The Chinese also meant the same by calling it *Chu She*. These names point towards the attractive property of the stone.

The magnetic stone found in mines is Ferric Oxide (FeO) out of which the artificial magnets are prepared. They are prepared by three methods:-

- Natural magnet is rubbed on the magnetic material, as a result of which the material is magnetised but has a low power.
- In the electrical method of magnetisation, an insulated wire is wound round the magnetic

substance and an electrical current is passed through the coil, for different periods of time to obtain different strengths. This process makes the magnet more powerful.

- Scientists have devised a machine called Magnetiser, which charges the magnetic material without using wires. It is being commonly used today to make artificial magnets and healing magnets.

What Makes the Nonmaterial into a Magnet?

The molecular theory explains the changes occurring in the nonmagnetic substance to magnetise it. As explained earlier, each atom is an individual magnet, but it is not capable of free existence. Therefore, it combines with other magnetic atoms to form molecules. Since they can exist independently, they become a single magnet. In a non-magnetised substance, the poles of all molecules do not point in one single direction, and are said to be misaligned. They lie jumbled up, thus the North Pole of one molecule neutralises the South Pole of the other, and therefore, does not show the properties of a magnet. The process of magnetisation gives direction to the molecules. All the molecules turn and move in one direction at one pole, i.e., at one end they face towards the north direction, while at the other they face towards the south, thus making the North

Pole and the South Pole respectively, and making a magnet out of it.

It is a physical change and the power of magnetisation depends upon the number of molecules pointing in the same direction at one end. The concentration of aligned molecules being maximum at the pole and minimum at the center.

This also explains the reason for the attraction of non-magnetised iron, which has its molecules all jumbled up. As the magnet is brought near this substance, the similar poles tend to move away, and the opposite poles of number of molecules get attracted and they pull the iron substance towards the magnet.

Every charged particle has two poles — North Pole and South Pole.

In a bar magnet, the poles are at opposite ends while in a circular magnet they are on opposite faces.

It is a universal law, 'Like poles repel each other and unlike poles attract each other'.

The force of attraction or repulsion depends upon the distance between them. Closer the poles, stronger is the force between them. Each particle or a piece broken from a bigger magnet will act as an independent magnet — may be permanent or temporary.

Magnetic field is the area in which the effect of the magnetic force or charge can be felt. It is represented by imaginary lines, which indicate the magnetic strength and direction. The magnetic strength is maximum at the poles.

The horseshoe is said to be magnetised and thus the horse can run so fast.

The Earth as a Magnet

Earth's Magnetism

The earth itself is considered as a huge magnet with its magnetic poles being in line and close to its geographical poles. This is the reason why the tiny compass needle always points towards the geographical North Pole.

All substances are made up of atoms. The outer sphere of these atoms has electrons. Every atom has an electrical charge: negative or positive, and it is the motion of electrons that create a magnetic field.

This makes each atom have its own magnetic field and force around it, which attracts other atoms. Thus, the atom has its own magnetic force besides the influence or impact of the earth's magnetic force. So, two types of magnetic energies act on each atom, cell or living being.

All human bodies are also enveloped in the magnetic field which has been termed as the astral body by the occultists. Man's vital, mental and physical health and its spiritual development is represented in the constitution of the invisible astral body or the magnetic field of the body.

The occultists have developed techniques to read the character and destiny, or to diagnose the patient's ailments by perceiving and decoding his astral aura.

According to this, every individual has a magnetic aura around their physical body which may be influenced by the aura of other bodies. That is the reason for liking or disliking an individual even before knowing him or her. The spiritual people exercise a deep impact on the consciousness of the common man when he comes in contact with them. This is because the magnetic field of such people are highly purified, strong, and occupy a greater range in space. Any evil thought present in the mind of common people of smaller magnetic strength, is eradicated by the stronger magnetic field. Similar is the case with physical illness also.

This is true Reiki treatment as well. When a healthy individual with a stronger magnetic field and energy touches the affected part of a patient or a weak individual, the transmission of energy takes place from the stronger to the weaker, and thus imparts curative energy required for healing the patient.

But we are here dealing with the physical ailment and disease, where magnet therapy has a role to play. This deals with the state when the sickness has transcended the vital and the mental level to the physical level. Here, the sickness exhibits symptoms and signs on the physical body, such as, pain, stiffness etc. Here we have subjective and objective symptoms to deal with. The human body is so weak that we have to give it magnetism in controlled quantities by creating artificial magnetic fields around permanent healing magnets.

The human body is constantly discharging emanations representing magnetism or electrical discharges. Electricity and magnetism are simultaneously produced in our body as they have the same basic energy, with a similar linked action. Magnetism is being produced by the body due to the presence of ferromagnetic substances in the body, like sodium, potassium, chlorine ions, iron, etc. Organs like the brain, heart, nerves, muscles and tissues create their own magnetic fields of different intensities. The strongest magnetic field is created by the human brain and that too, during sleep.

These magnetic fields fluctuate with the changing mind of the individual and change in the physical environment inside the body. These fluctuations are instantly reflected in the astral body. Scientists have made devices and instruments to measure the fluctuating magnetic fields of individual organs — heart, brain, lungs, muscles and so on. Maximum magnetic field is produced by the brain — 10^8 gauss and heart — 10^7 gauss.

Magnet therapy helps to maintain the equilibrium of magnetic fields inside the body with the help of man-made magnets.

Substances or materials that carry many atomic dipoles are called ferromagnetic, such as Lodestone etc. These also constitute magnetic ores. If these substances are touched by a permanent magnet, they can be charged permanently. This is how we prepare permanent healing magnets, which are used in medical treatment.

Magnetic Energy

All the energies are generally derived from the sun. It is believed that with the sun as the main source, the objects could not get away from its force of attraction and kept on revolving around it in their orbits. They are called planets. The earth is one of the planets. It possesses a bipolar magnet, with its magnetic poles coinciding with the geographical poles.

There is a slight contradiction about this theory. Some people believe that the earth has opposite magnetism, i.e., the South Pole at geographical North Pole and the North Pole at geographical South Pole. But it is not so, because the poles are named according to the magnetic needle pointing towards them. According to the new school of thought, the magnetic pole coincides with the geographical poles of the earth.

This planet (earth) exerts some force of attraction on each and every object. This force of attraction is called the gravitational force. Each object is made up of molecules and atoms. In every atom, there is a nucleus that contains protons, neutrons and electrons that constantly move in a fixed orbit around the nucleus. There is a magnetic attraction between the nucleus, the protons which are positively charged and the electrons which are negatively charged. This is the same configuration as the universe. This force of attraction, within the object itself and among different objects, is called the magnetic force or magnetic energy.

It is believed that all objects on the earth possess a magnetic energy of its own due to which it maintains its existence on the earth. Also, the external environment and the atmosphere influence it. Here, the external forces of other energies or other bodies acting as individual magnets attract it. This helps to maintain its position and relationship with the surrounding objects. We have certain instruments that can measure the magnetic power of each substance. It is this energy that we use for healing purpose.

What Is an Illness?

Before we discuss an illness, I want to emphasise on normal health — What is it that gives us life?

In a dead body, the cells, the organs, the whole anatomy of an individual is intact. Then what is it that is absent? Is it the soul? Is it the force, or is it the vital energy?

Yes, vital energy seems to be the most appropriate answer. It is this energy that is withdrawn from the cells that is responsible for its death. It is this energy which is responsible for normal functioning of the cells and, in turn, the human system. This energy gives life to the whole system. It is derived from the mother's womb initially, then from the food we eat and drink, the atmosphere, i.e., the air we breathe, and above all the biggest source of energy, the sun. Like plants, we also derive a major part of our energy from the sun.

A harmonious flow of energy leads to a healthy life. When this harmony is disturbed due to external factors, the cells or the system become low on energy. This is when the functioning of organs becomes impaired and the body starts feeling low and tired.

Animals and plants are more close to nature and respond to bodily needs and go into hibernation so that they do not fall sick. Once the energy level is restored, they lead a normal life. But human beings are leading a very stressful life. In today's lifestyle, they are continuously running after material things. In the process, they have gone against nature and more so away from it. To the extent we are also trying to convert nature as per their requirements. Cutting forests, bringing down mountains, building houses and factories, killing animals, turning the course of rivers as per their requirements, building dams to stop or control the natural water, etc, are all examples of changing nature to suit their requirements.

Human beings today are living in an artificial environment, and leading an artificial life surrounded by machines. They are eating synthetic food, in the form of tablets and powders. As a result they become weak and fall sick. Health does not survive in an artificial environment.

In an individual there is no life without energy. It is this vital energy that is required to maintain the normal functioning of the body. Now due to some factors like late nights, eating rich or fried food, excessive tension on mind, or bad news or shocks or any unwanted situation in daily life, cause sudden lowering of vital energies. If not paid attention, then the energy level falls to such an extent that it hampers the normal functioning of the body, thereby lowering the immunity or resistance of the individual. This is the stage when the person suffers from the disease at the functional level. At this stage, although there are no signs of any particular disease, the individual shows certain symptoms. There is a feeling of general discomfort. Many of us sometimes experience sudden backache, headache or lethargy, without having done much work. All these symptoms are indicators of the body's call for rest, as it feels exhausted. This is the stage of low vitality and the period when the individual is susceptible to diseases. If still the person carries on, and does not rest, the energy level falls further and develops into a pathological disease.

It is at this stage that investigations start and there are signs of a disease. It is now that doctors can recognise the disease. It is important to know that everyone is born with certain susceptibility towards a system. It is here that he exhibits his symptoms first, hence the family history will tell us where to look for the diseases in an individual, if the patient comes to us in the predecease stage.

Now, in all the stages stated above, we have seen that it is only the energy level in the body that has changed from one stage to another in the body. It is energy that is responsible for normal functioning of the body. The energy, when withdrawn from a system, disturbs its normal functioning. Energy when further withdrawn from an organ, alters its functioning, in the form of an infection or growth.

It is observed that when the energy level is lowered, it becomes easy for the bacteria or the virus to attack and cause illness. Therefore, its treatment can be done by energy-giving products only. A magnet is one of them. They may not be curative at the drastic pathological level but can certainly aid in providing the energy to fight the disease, i.e., to enhance the production of curative energy in the body.

The magnetic energy so provided by creating a local magnetic field around the affected area gives some relief to the patient. If the disease is at the functional level, magnetic energy alone can prove curative.

It is believed that every human body has its own curative energy. This, when lowered, results in sickness. Thus for the purpose of curing, this low energy has to be replaced either by magnets, diathermy, yoga or meditation, or by homeopathic doses.

How Do Magnets Help in Sickness?

Magnets are a source of natural energy and thus aid in giving us energy so required in the artificial environment. Regular use of magnet therapy boosts our immune system and help us live a healthy life. After having understood how and why we fall sick, the treatment becomes easier.

It should be understood that we fall sick due to internal weakness, that allows the external factors like bacteria or virus to enter our body and create havoc. If this is so, then medicines like antibiotics or antiviral alone cannot cure. For a complete cure, we have to build our energy levels to the optimum level so that the external negative factors cannot enter or affect our body.

We fall sick because the energy level in a particular organ lowers. When we apply magnets to that region, it helps in two ways:-

- It attracts the iron salts in the blood and thus improves the local circulation, hence treating any inflammation, swelling, stiffness, pains, etc.

- The bipolar magnets so applied in the region create a magnetic field of their own, and impart the correct amount of positive energy required for healing. This combats for the low energy also and makes the body strong and healthy.

However, it does not mean that medicines are not required at all, but in some cases where the sickness is at a pathological level, and the bacterial infection has set in, there magnetic energy is given along with oral medicines. While the medicines take care of the infection, the magnets look after the low vitality, thus imparting complete cure for the ailment.

There is another factor made out of magnets, i.e., magnetised water. This is used to purify the blood. It also acts as a diuretic, and helps in urinary infections, renal or ureteric calculus, renal diseases, and renal failure. Even in generalised oedema it is very useful, as it is a diuretic.

It also helps in lowering the blood pressure indirectly. For high blood pressure there are certain wristbands or belts which are tied on the left wrist to lower the pressure while on the right wrist to increase the low pressure.

There is also a necklace for dealing with respiratory and cardiac problems. It helps in improving the local blood circulation in the heart and lungs. It prevents clotting in the cardiac arteries, or phlegm formation in the lungs. It has also been observed that magnets can treat 40 to 50 per cent of coronary blockage.

The latest use of magnets is in the form of small magnets of button size. These small magnets are extremely powerful. They are applied on the acupressure points of the affected organs, and also on the palm or on the foot. They prove to be much more effective and powerful than the high power magnets. The action of the magnets is through nerves rather than physical.

Magnetic Appliances

Following are some magnetic appliances used in magnet therapy:-

- High power magnet pair of 3000 gauss power – This is used to treat almost all pains.
- Premier pair of magnets of 1500 gauss power – This is used for treating neurological problems. It is effective in giving intense penetrating magnetic waves.
- Low power ceramic magnets of 300 gauss power – These are used for application near the brain region. It is used for improving eyesight, treating cataract, glaucoma and other retinal problems. It is also helpful in increasing height in children. It is used to treat headaches and migraines.
- Lumbar spondylitic belt — It is used to treat lumbar spondylitis, slip disc, disc prolapsed, lumbage, etc, and to a certain extent, reduces extra fat on the abdomen, when the magnet area is placed in front.

- Cervical collar or belt — This is used in cases of cervical spondylitis. It helps the studying children because they sit and write continuously for long hours, and strain their neck muscles, a pre-stage of spondylosis.
- Wristbands — They are in the form of beautiful bracelets. They are used to treat high or low blood pressure at initial stages, and improve the blood circulation.
- Necklaces — These are used to keep the chest in perfect health, especially the heart and lungs.
- Button magnets — These are Japanese magnets of very small size. They are fixed to the sole of the shoe or taped to the skin on the acupressure points to give the desired result without actually puncturing with the needle. These are also seen to be very effective in various other diseases and seem to be opening new domains of treatment by magnetism.

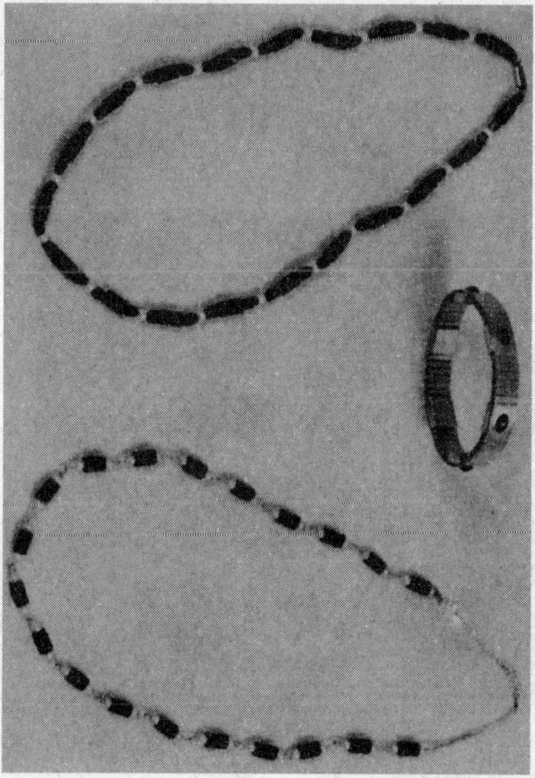

Necklace and wristband

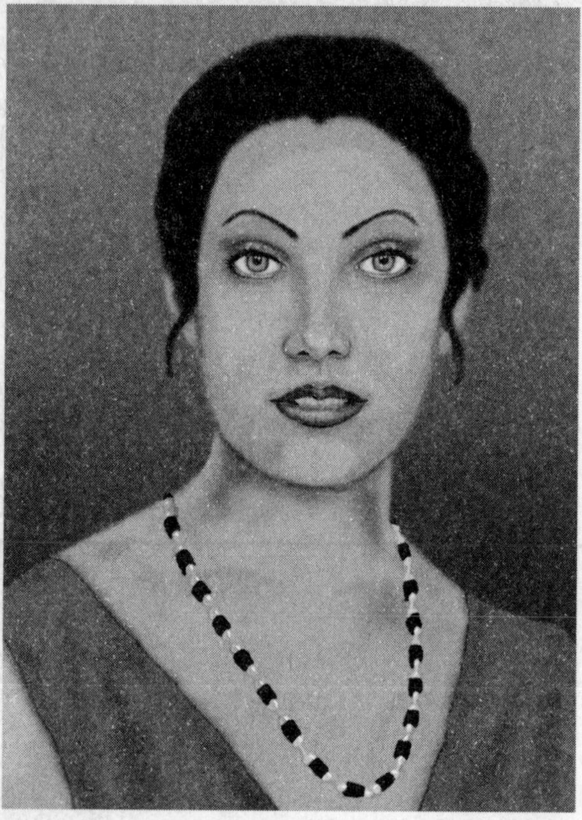

Necklace

- Magnetised water — This is prepared by keeping the water on each pole of high power magnets for 12 to 24 hours. After this, the water of two poles is mixed and then used for drinking purpose. It is an effective diuretic and a blood cleanser.
- Magnetised oil — Any oil is magnetised by keeping it on the magnets for 12 to 24 hours. It is very effective for dandruff, falling of hair and premature greying of hair.

Limitations of Magnetism

It is important to note that just everybody cannot tolerate the effects of magnetism. There are people who are very sensitive to magnetism and may react to the therapy.

- Sometimes people experience an increase in the pulse rate.
- The application of magnet may lead to an increase in the body heat, or tachycardia, or sometimes vertigo also. This is due to sudden rush of blood to these areas.
- Another word of caution is that magnetic treatment is an aid to treating, in the alternative systems. It is not always curative in itself. As stated earlier, it depends upon the stage of the disease. Only diseases at the functional level come under its domain. Other diseases are helped by magnets in treatment but can be cured with medicines of any system.

Homeopathy goes very well with magnet therapy, as the purpose of treatment in both is the same, i.e., balancing the energy levels in the body. Both treat the patients by increasing the curative power of the individual. It is interesting to know that we have three medicines prepared from magnetism in homeopathy.

Moreover, the physician should not be too optimistic and must evaluate the case from time to time. It is important to observe whether the patient is actually healing, or is just being palliated by the treatment. The physician should also observe if the disease is not being transferred from one organ to the other.

Diseases and Magnet Therapy

Magnet therapy means treatment done by the magnets specifically designed for healing. Channelling body's own curative force and providing for the low energy levels that is the main cause of sickness, even if the individual is taking some medication for the disease, the actual loss of energy is repaired by the magnets.

Naturopathy also helps by replacing the energy loss through mud, air, and sunlight, while magnet therapy replenishes the loss by permanent healing magnets.

The most common diseases that fall in the domain of the treatment of magnet therapy are orthopaedic and neurological diseases. Circulatory problems also, to a certain extent, can be treated by magnet therapy but one also has to take medicines.

Pains, aches, swellings, stiffness, joint problems, paralytic disorders, neuralgia, ureteric calculus, sprains, etc, are effectively treated by this system of alternative medicine.

Magnets can be applied to any system of medicine. It does not contradict, on the contrary, helps the medicines to heal faster by accelerating their action, and also provide for the low energy which the medicines are not able to.

Magnet therapy forms a part of Naturopathy, i.e., the treatment through nature's laws. Magnet therapy is easy to do and is the simplest form of external treatment. It is also quite cheap and can be afforded by anybody. A pair of magnetic set so purchased by a family proves to be useful for all members, and not only for the treatment but also for a healthy living. A pair of magnets can be used for a number of ailments. Once purchased, the magnets are permanent and do not lose their power if properly kept.

In today's world, everyone is so busy and running short of time, that by evening or night when they return home they are dead tired. Magnetic application for only ten minutes will put in more life into you and will also prevent you from so many diseases that may find a place in your body because of a stressful life you are leading.

Magnet therapy also cures nervous or physical exhaustion in an individual. By giving energy, it also charges and freshens up all the systems, so that he/she starts looking fresh and charming, young and ready for the next job. It has been observed that regular use of magnets retards the ageing process. Isn't that interesting? All of us do want to remain young for ever.

Above all, the magnets do not produce any side-effects on our body by creating new complications, like the modern medicines do. Of course, if applied for too long, in some cases it can produce slight tachycardia, tiredness, and diuresis. But as this is very short-lived, it wears off once the body is withdrawn from the application.

Types of Magnets

The healing magnets, and magnetised water are available to us for treating various ailments or diseases :—

1. HP — High Power Magnets, 3000 gauss power
2. MP — Medium Power Magnets, 1500 gauss power
3. LP — Low Power Magnets, 500 gauss power
4. MW — Magnetised Water, dosage — 2 ounces/ 3 to 4 times a day for adults.
5. MWN — Magnetised Water of North Pole
6. MWS — Magnetised Water of South Pole

Uses of Magnetised Water

Magnetic water's efficacy is best observed in the digestive system, urinary system and nervous system.

Digestive System

Magnetic water treats constipation and its related problems, the commonest being hyperacidity. It also reduces excess bile, and retching, etc. It improves the functioning of the liver.

- By improving the basic ailment, i.e., constipation, it helps to expel the toxins of the body and prevents accumulation of poisonous substances in the body. Thus, by cleansing the digestive tract, it improves appetite and digestion of the food. It gives more energy and health to the suffering body. Also, by improving digestion and the functioning of liver, it helps indirectly to treat allergies, like asthma, bronchitis, cold and cough, skin allergies, etc.

Nervous System

Magnetised water soothes the nerves and has a sedative effect.

- In nervous disorders, it helps to increase low blood pressure.
- It also helps to clear the blocked blood vessels, if any, and increases and improves the blood circulation to the brain.
- It removes depression and mental exhaustion at the end of the day.
- Magnetised water improves eyesight, eye infections, wounds, conjunctivitis, etc by washing the affected parts two to three times a day.
- Swellings and inflammations are also checked by washing the part with magnetised water several times a day.

Urinary System

Magnetised water taken orally acts as a diuretic. Hence, it helps in expulsion of stone or calculus present in the kidney or ureter.

- If the stone is in the bladder, a cup of magnetised water if taken every two hours and exercises after that will expel the stone faster.
- It is also effective in chronic urinary tract infections.
- Being a diuretic, magnetised water also helps in lowering high blood pressure and oedema of the body.

Types of Magnetised Water

Magnetised water is of three varieties — the bipolar MW, the North Pole MW, and the South Pole MW

The Bipolar Magnetised Water

It is prepared by keeping water in two glass bottles on two HP magnet for 24 hours. Then the two waters so charged are mixed together before use. This is called bipolar magnetised water.

- It is best to treat the general complaints of indigestion or urinary diseases.

The North Pole Magnetised Water

A bottle of water is kept only on the high power North Pole and after 24 hours, it is ready for use.

- It is most effective in treating infections in the body, internally as well as externally.
- It is also helpful in treatment of eczema with secondary infections, urinary tract infections, ulcers, etc, because it inhibits the formation or

growth of bacteria and helps in curing the infection.

The South Pole Magnetised Water

A bottle of water is kept on the South Pole for 24 hours.

- It is effective in treating abcess, boils, viral infections, etc, as this promotes the growth of bacteria. In an abcess, it is desired to let it grow first so that no infection is left inside, and then it bursts on its own. MWSP is given orally and the area is washed externally with it as well.
- It is effective in sty of the eye, foreign body in eye, and skin abcess, etc.

It is known that the two poles of a permanent magnet have different roles to play in the healing process. In fact it was Dr Hanemann, a German physicist and the founder of homeopathy, who discovered it. He made three medicines out of magnets and studied the different effects of the two poles separately.

Effects of the North Pole

- The North Pole has more affinity for the right side of the body and the front or the ventral side of the body.
- The North Pole magnet is effective in treating diseases caused by infections such as arthritis, boils, skin eczema, wounds, ear infections, toothaches, pyorrhoea, caries of teeth, cancer, ulcers, tumors, urinary infections, tonsillitis, etc.
- North Pole reduces the growth of bacteria and removes the swelling and inflammation.
- It may be applied locally at the site of infection or given orally in the form of MWNP.

Effects of the South Pole

- The South Pole has more affinity for the left side or back of the body.
- It helps to treat the pains of all kinds and acts as an analgesic without any side-effects.

- It is effective in neuralgia, stiffness, paralytic or paretic conditions, weakness of any kind. It also helps in curing functional disorders like gas formation, indigestion, heart ailments, circulatory defects, etc.

In application, since the effect of two poles is different, we have two theories of application — the unipolar theory of application and the bipolar theory of application.

Unipolar theory is used only for treating specific diseases and not general diseases. Since it does not create a magnetic field of its own it is not so effective.

Therefore, the bipolar theory of application is more widely accepted and used in treatment.

Like in electropathy, the circuit is complete only when both poles are applied simultaneously, similarly in magnet therapy, the desired results are obtained only when the circuit is completed by applying both the poles together. Then only will it produce its own magnetic field and thus provide the sick body with additional energy required for healing and curing.

Types of Treatment by Magnet Therapy

The treatment by magnets is divided into two categories:

1. Local Treatment
2. General Treatment

Local Treatment

- Here the selected pole is applied on the diseased area. The magnetic pole is to touch on the affected part of the body, without applying any pressure on it. If the discase falls in the infective group, the North Pole is applied. If the disease is functional or inflammatory, the South Pole is applied.
- If it is thought that both poles are required, then the North Pole is applied on the right, upper, or front side of the body while the South Pole is applied on the left, lower or dorsal of the body, simultaneously.
- The power of the magnet is chosen according to the strength of the ailment and the capacity of the patient.

The instruments used for local treatment are:—

- High power magnets
- Medium power magnets
- Low power magnets
- Premier pair of bipolar magnets
- Necklace for chest ailments
- Cervical spondylosis belt
- Lumbar belt
- Knee cap for knee arthritis
- Wristbands for hypertension
- Head belt for migraines and headaches
- Small button magnets for application on acupressure points.

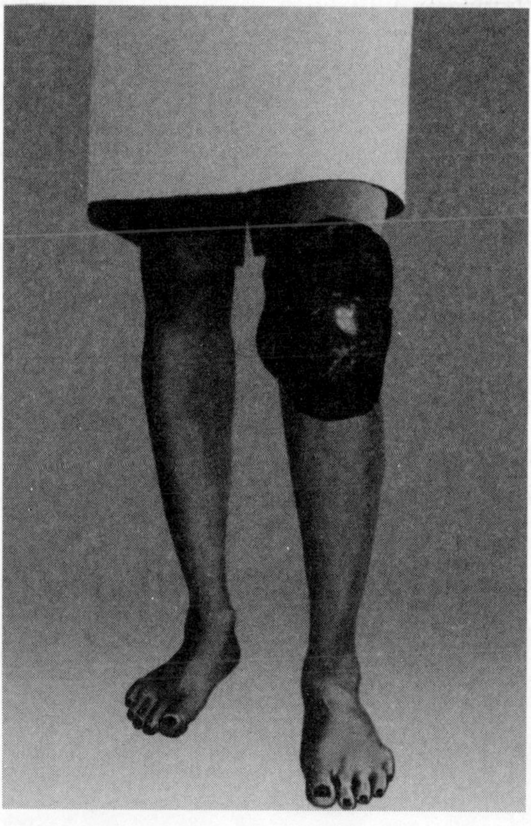

Knee cap for knee arthritis

General Treatment

- When the ailment or the disease is not localised to a particular organ or area, for instance systemic diseases, like diabetes, urinary tract infection, general malaise, etc, the magnets are applied under the soles or palms. The soles and palms are linked with the heart and brain and to almost all parts of the body, so they are chosen to give general treatment.

In the following pages we have described the five methods of applying magnets in order to cover all organs of the body.

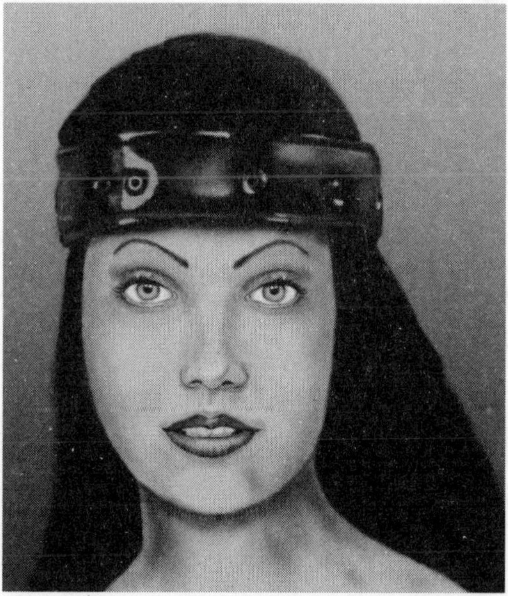

Head belt for headaches, migraines and insomnia

a) **Method 1**

- This is used for treating diseases of upper half of the body.
- The right palm is placed on the North Pole magnet while the left palm on the South Pole magnet for 10 to 30 minutes.
- It treats arthritis of the hands, stiff neck, chest ailments like asthma, bronchitis, heart diseases, etc.

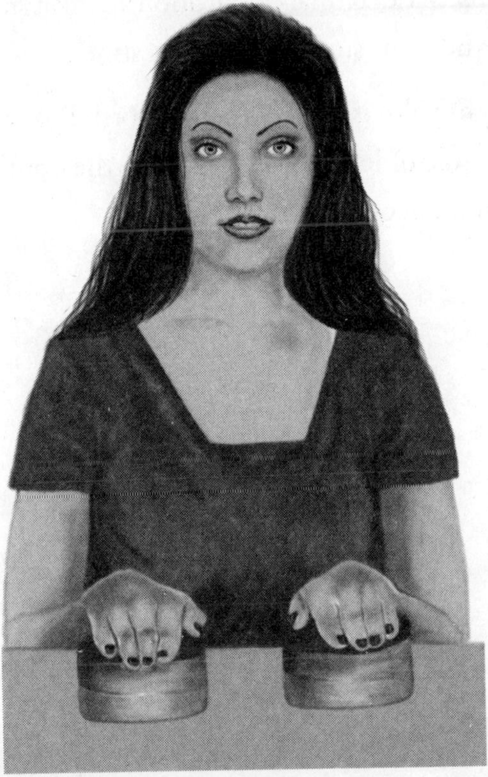

Method 1

b) **Method 2**

- This is a diagonal application to treat ailments of the liver, stomach and intestines.
- Right palm is placed on the North Pole whereas the sole of left foot is placed on the South Pole, simultaneously.

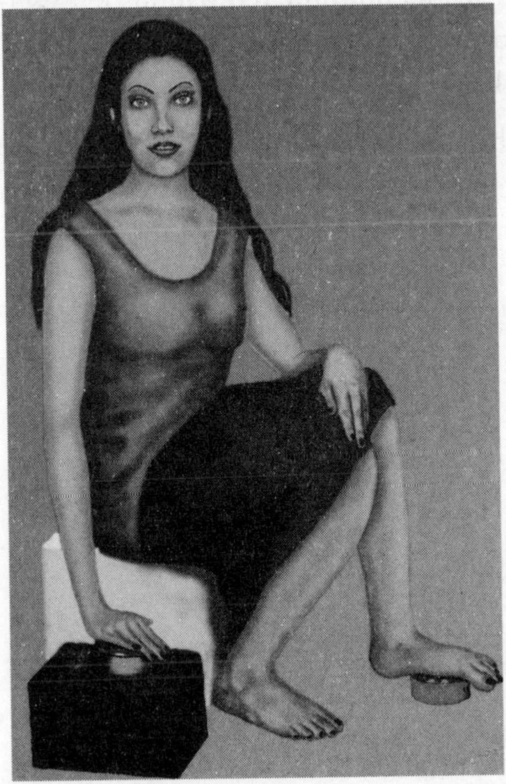

Method 2

c) **Method 3**

- In this method the left palm is placed on the North Pole and the sole of left foot on the South Pole.
- It helps in curing left side ailments like paralysis, stroke of the left side, polio, etc.

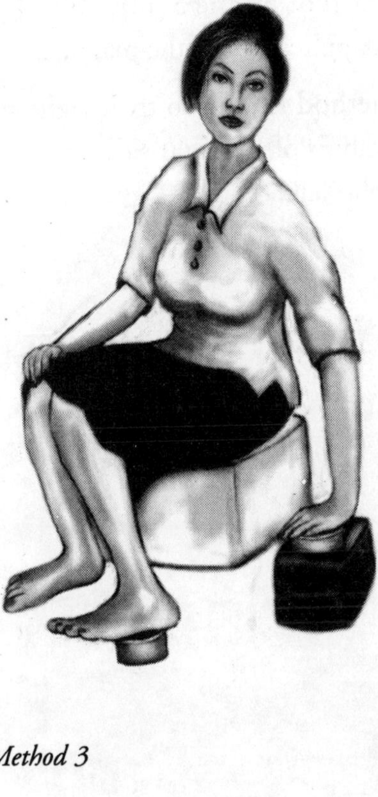

Method 3

d) **Method 4**

- The right palm is placed on the North Pole with the right foot on the South Pole. This is called vertical application of the magnets.
- This method is used to treat right side diseases like paralysis of the right side, stroke of the right side, polio, etc.

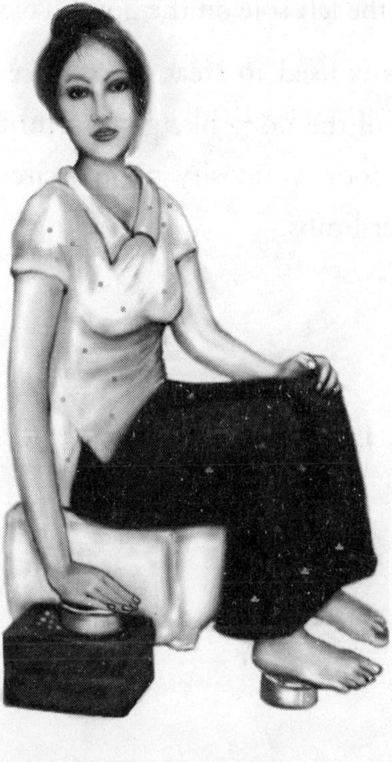

Method 4

e) **Method 5**

- The right foot sole is placed on the North Pole and the left sole on the South Pole.
- This is used to treat the diseases of the lower half of the body like gout, arthritis of the knee and foot, varicosity or low circulation to the lower limbs.

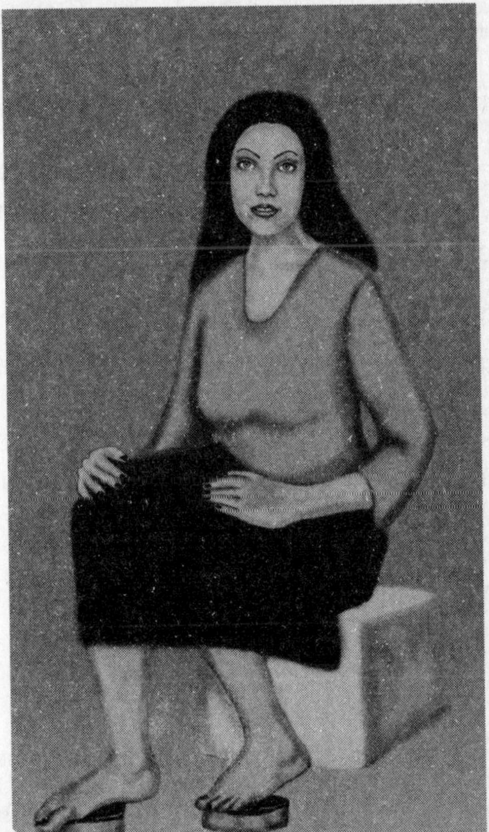

Method 5

Precautions to Be Observed During the Treatment

- Time of treatment — Morning, after bath and before breakfast.
- Cold food and drinks should not be taken for an hour after applying HP magnets. Warm and hot things can be taken after the application to maintain the warmth generated by the magnetic application.
- Bath, swimming or exposure to cold water should be avoided after the application.
- H P or M P magnets should not be applied immediately after meals. It may lead to nausea or vomiting in some cases.
- Pregnant women, weak and sensitive women and children should not use high power magnets. They can use upto 1500 gauss power magnets.
- High power magnets should not be applied to the eyes, head or heart areas of the body.

- Watches should be kept away from the field of magnets.
- High power magnets should not be used for too long a period. It may lead to heaviness in the head, increased sleepiness, tingling sensation in the nerves, etc. However, if such symptoms are observed in a patient after application, the doctor should be consulted, and the patient should take rest. Homeopathic medicine like, Zinc Met 30 may be taken as an antidote.
- If the wrong pole is applied for long, it may be antidoted by keeping the palms on a zinc plate or the medicine-Zinc Met 6 or 30 can be taken.
- When the H P and M P magnets are not being used, they are kept joined with a keeper between the two poles so that magnetism is not wasted, or the magnets are not demagnetised.
- While taking treatment with H P or M P magnets, one should sit on a wooden plank to cut oneself off from the earth's magnetic power.

Diseases to Be Treated by Magnet Therapy

Arthritis

- This is a disease of the joints.
- It is characterised by stiffness of the joints, pain in the joints, swelling in the joints with local heat which may or may not be followed by lack of movement of the joint.
- This disease may be localised to one joint or may be a systemic application of the disease where all the joints may be affected.
- The different types of arthritis known to us today are — rheumatoid arthritis, osteoarthritis periarthritis.

Rheumatoid Arthritis

- Here the stiffness of the joint is caused by fluid collection in the joint space.

- The affected joint swells, is red and hot to touch, with lack of movement. It is also inflamed.
- The joints gets deformed, and moves away from the medial plain of the body.
- There is a spindle-shaped swelling of the joint.

Treatment

- Magnet application helps in treating the inflammation of the joint and thus reducing the swelling and stiffness of the joint.
- The South Pole is placed on a wooden board, the affected joint is placed on the magnet and the North Pole is placed on the upper part of the joint, for at least 10 minutes in the morning and 10 minutes in the evening for 15 days.
- The time span of application may be increased by a minute every day reaching upto 20 minutes at one go.

Osteoarthritis

- Here there is generally no inflammation but the joint space is reduced due to extra or excessive calcium deposits in the joint, thus causing stiffness and lack of movement of the joint.
- First joint to be affected is the knee joint as it is the weight-bearing joint.
- The patient experiences stiffness in the knee and is unable to walk freely, especially in the mornings, or on first movement.
- The patient also feels difficulty in bending or stretching the knees. The larger joints are generally the first ones to be affected.
- The major difficulty experienced by the patient is in bending the joint, or on climbing and coming down the stairs, as the deposits reduce the joint space.

Treatment

- For knees, there are special belts made of low power magnets. They are tied on the joint and the patient sits for 30 to 40 minutes, once a day.

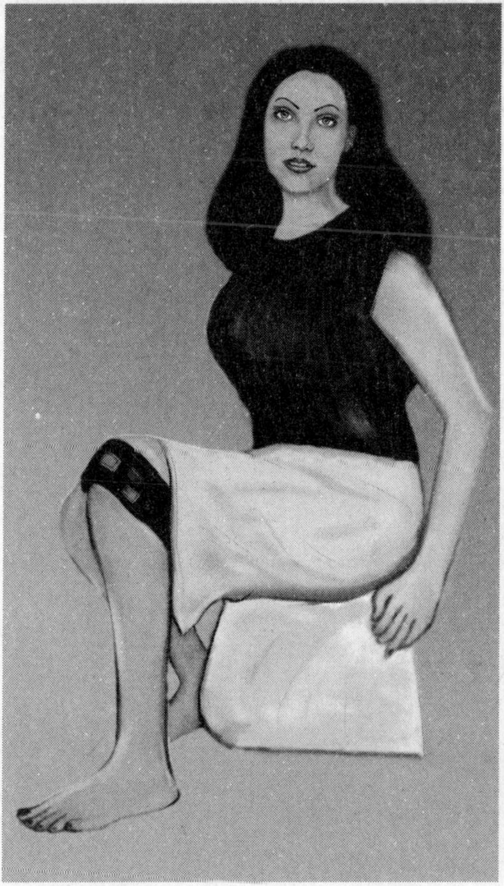

Osteoarthritis

- The high power of magnets also help to dissolve the extra deposit of calcium.
- The South Pole of high power magnet is placed on the bed or a wooden stool and the knee is placed on it facing upwards.

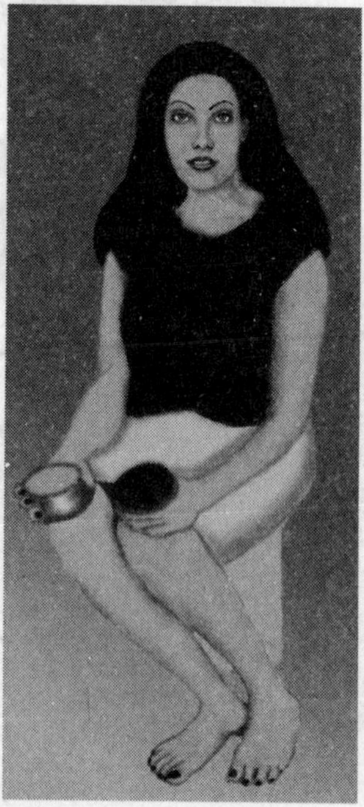

Osteoarthritis

- The North Pole is then placed on top of it for 10 minutes and gradually increased upto 20 minutes, twice a day for one month in order to get favourable results.

Periarthritis

- Tendonitis, sinovitis, or inflammation of the surrounding areas of the joints cause stiffness of the affected areas.

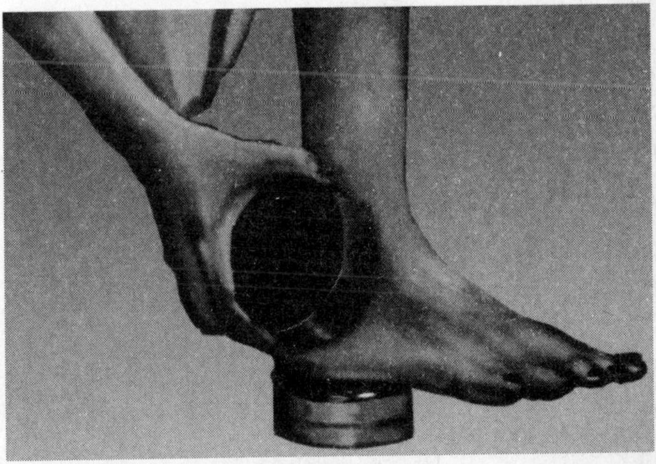

Ankle arthritis

- Generally there is no inflammation or infection of the joint.

Treatment

- The South Pole is placed under the affected joint and the North Pole on the upper surface of the joint.
- This application increases the local blood supply to the joint.

Injury to the Joints and Magnet Therapy

Sprains

- When any particular muscle gets pulled or injured and goes into a spasm, i.e., becomes stiff and any movement of that joint becomes painful and impossible, it is said to be sprained.

Treatment

- An increase in the blood supply to the local sprained area is the solution, whether it is done by giving hot fomentation or by applying magnets to that area.
- Magnets here help in two ways, firstly, they increase the local blood circulation by attracting the Iron (Fe_2) of the blood, and secondly, they create a local magnetic field around that joint and thus help in relieving the pain as well as the stiffness. Hence, it helps the muscle to get rid of the spasm or sprain.

Sports Injury

- This is the major topic of concern today because of the increasing interest in sports all over the world.
- This includes orthopaedic injuries such as tendovitis, sprain, fractures, stiffness of muscles, slip disc, ruptured muscles, spondylosis — cervical or lumbar.
- It also includes neurological injuries like paresis, lower motor neuron diseases, paralysis of any particular area, Ryter's syndrome in comatose patients where the cause is internal haemorrhage or a clot formation.
- The premier pair of bipolar magnets are best in treating such injuries.
- Here the magnetism is deep penetrating and longer lasting or gives a more sustaining effect.
- The South Pole is applied under the joint and the North Pole on the upper part of the joint.

- In case of neurological injuries, the magnets are applied vertically. The North Pole is applied at a higher position on the body that is towards the head, while the South Pole is applied on the lower end of the body, i.e., towards the legs.
- If the injury has caused a slip disc and the numbness or pain is there in the right lower limb, the North Pole is applied on the lower back in the lumbosacral area while the South Pole is applied on the back of the knee joint or to the point upto where the numbness extends.
- In cases of clot formations or haemorrhages, magnets help in the formation of collateral blood vessels to combat the need of the organ.

Treatment of Spondylosis by Magnet Therapy

Cervical Spondylosis

- In this ailment, the disc spaces get narrowed and apply pressure on the nerves.
- This may be due to osteoarthritis or wrong curvature of the spine or wrong posture while working, or due to prolonged sitting and working.

Symptoms

- Pain in the nape of neck, which may extend even to the arm or fingers. At times, it may resemble angina pain. It may be associated with numbness and become worse on hanging the limb downwards.
- Vertigo
- Headaches

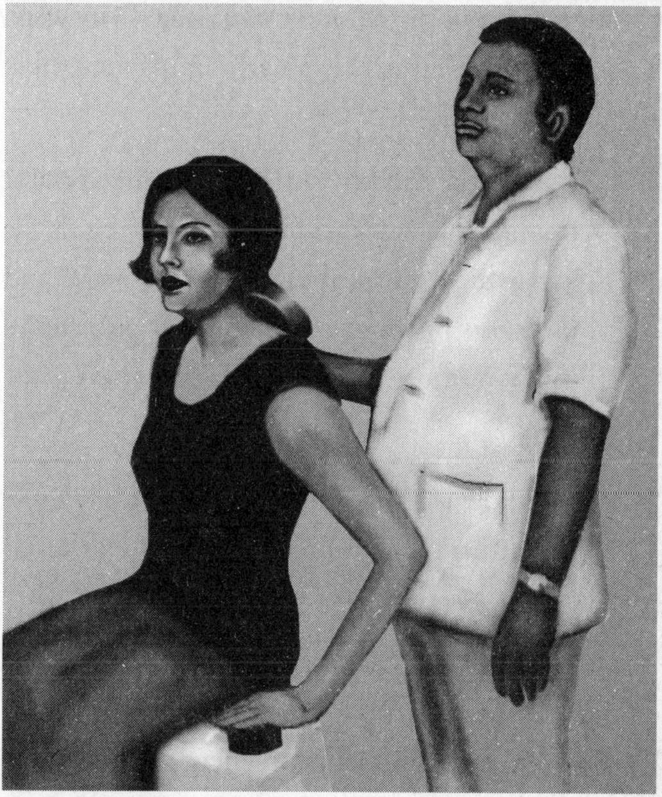

Cervical spondylosis

- Pain or numbness in the shoulders or even extending upto the outer two fingers, in some cases, if present in the left arm, it may resemble a heart attack.

  Diagnosis is done by an X-ray of the cervical vertebrae, that shows minimal narrowing of the spaces which puts a pressure on the nerve and thus causes the above symptoms. It also shows formation of osteophytes in the vertebrae.

Treatment

- North Pole is applied at the nape of neck while the South Pole is applied below the affected hand.

- There is also a cervical collar belt that can be tied around the neck. It supports the neck and also gives it the magnetic energy required for smooth functioning.

Lumbar Spondylosis

- A lumbar belt is used for curing this condition. The lumbar belt has low power magnets in the region of lumbar vertebrae.

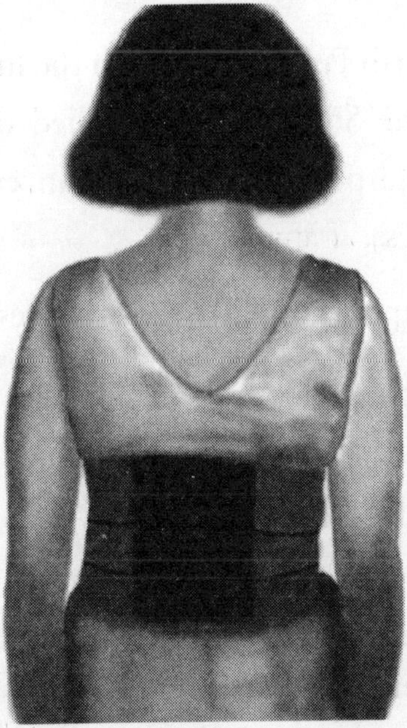

Lumbar spondylosis

- It is characterised by occurrence of spondylosis in the lumbar region.

Treatment

- This is treated by using a lumbar belt or using high power magnets.
- The North Pole is applied on the lumbar region while the South Pole is applied on the lower limb, the point where the pain extends to or numbness, if any.
- This is applied for 20 to 30 minutes, twice daily.

Slip Disc

- Lumbar belt helps to give support to the back and treats stiffness also.
- We use the North Pole on the upper end of the numb area and the South Pole on the lower end of the numb area for 10-20 minutes.

Lumbago

- It is a backache in the lumbosacral region or in the lumbar region.

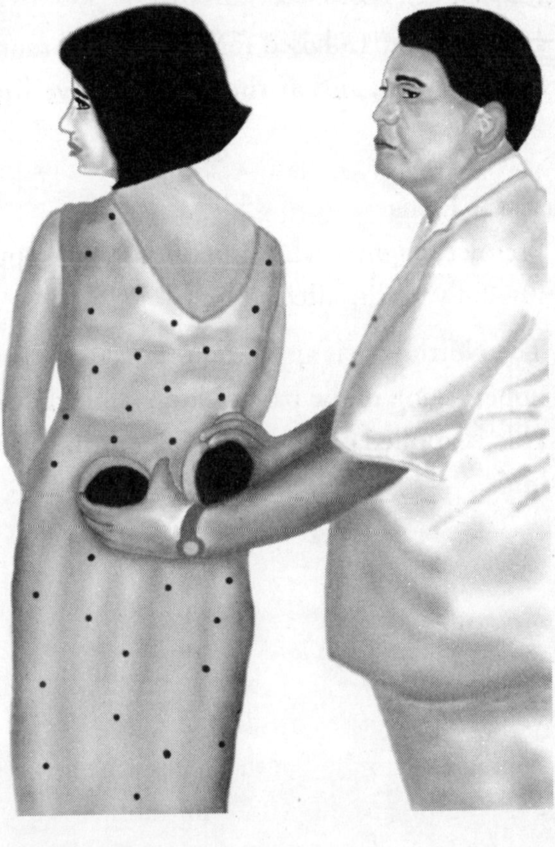

Lumbar spondylosis

Treatment

- Lumbar belt is advised for 30 minutes, morning and evening, and at the time of travelling or exertion.

Muscular Pains

- Premier magnets which are bipolar, are applied vertically on the affected limbs.
- The North Pole is applied on the shoulder or the upper region of the painful limb while the South Pole is applied on the lower area of the affected limb.

Treatment of other diseases by Magnet Therapy

Gangrene

- This is another sphere where magnets have a great deal to offer.
- The North pole is applied on the upper surface of the gangrenous area while the South Pole is applied on the lower surface for 15 minutes, twice daily, to improve the blood circulation.
- High power magnets are best suited for this condition.

Chilblains

- This is a winter problem. Here the feet, toes, fingers or hands become cold and swollen due to lack of blood supply to the periphery.
- There is a lot of itching in the toes.

Treatment

- The North Pole of high power magnets is placed below the right toes and the South Pole below the left toes for 15 minutes, twice daily.

Stroke (Hemiplegia)

- This is a condition of nerve paralysis caused by lack of blood supply to a particular area of the brain.
- In this, half side of the body becomes paralysed.
- Generally it is motor paralysis and the sensations are intact.

Treatment

- The North Pole of high power magnet is placed under the right palm and the South Pole under the left palm for 10 minutes.
- The North Pole of high power magnet is placed under the right sole and the South Pole under the left sole for 10 minutes.
- The North Pole of high power is placed under the affected side palm and the South Pole under the same side sole for 10 minutes.

All these three exercises are to be repeated twice daily, along with physiotherapy.

Lower Motor Neuron Disease

- In this ailment, a single limb gets paralysed due to injury disc displacement. It may be motor and sensory both, or simple foot drop also.

Treatment

- Premier pair of magnets is used.
- The North Pole is placed on the spine in between the shoulders in case of upper limb and on lumbar region in case of lower limb, while the South Pole is placed under the palm or on the sole of the affected limb for 20 minutes everyday.

Kidney Diseases

- Nephritis, renal calculus, ureteric calculus, recurrent urinary infections fall under this domain.

Treatment

- Here instead of application of magnets, magnetised water has a greater role to play.
- Being a diuretic, magnetised water helps to wash out the toxins from the system easily.
- We have seen ureteric calculus passing out only with magnetised water, without any medication.

Blood Pressure

- High blood pressure, without any pathology, can be controlled to a great extent by wearing the wristband or the bracelet on the left wrist.
- The same band on the right wrist treats low blood pressure.

Several beautiful wristbands made in silver and magnets for women are available which have proved their efficacy in treating high blood pressure.

Magnets are useful not only in treating high BP but also its after effects, like on kidneys, stroke, or clot formation, etc.

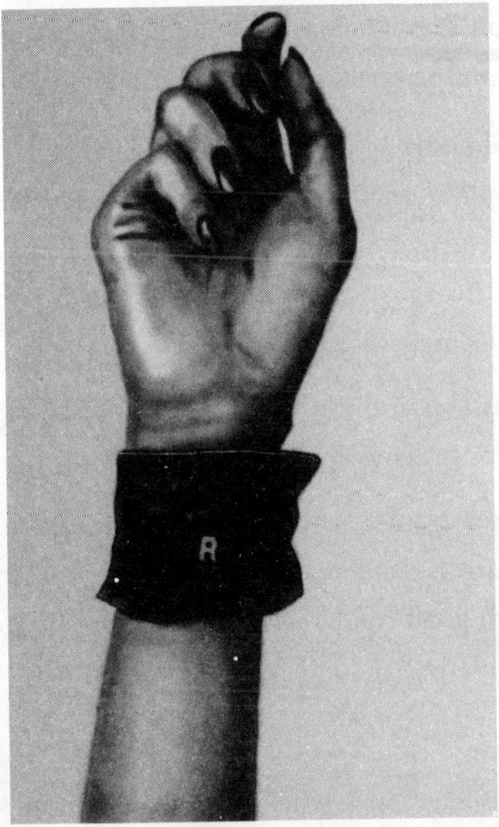

High blood pressure

Magnetised water is also used in the treatment of high BP, as it helps in the circulation, purifies the blood and removes or rather dissolves the clots.

Eye Ailments

- Application of low power magnets, i.e., crescent type magnets on the eyes for 15 minutes in the morning and 15 minutes in the evening immensely improves the eyesight.
- Washing of the eyes with magnetised water also helps in removing the tiredness of the eyes.
- Diseases of eyes like myopia, hypermetropia, cataract, glaucoma, conjunctivitis, etc are treated with good results in magnet therapy, if applied regularly.

Sinusitis

- This is a disease where there is mucus collection in the inside space, around the nose and eyes.
- There are maxillary sinus and the frontal sinus. These get blocked due to mucus collection.

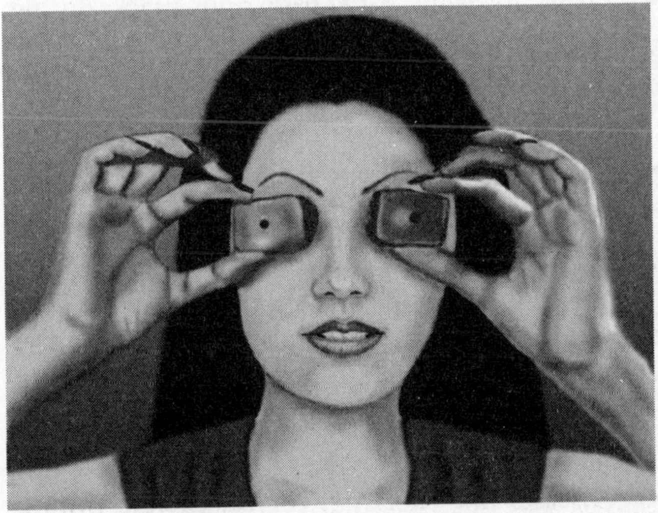

Eye ailments

- This causes headaches, and blockage of the nose, also difficulty in breathing especially while lying down.
- Generally people suffer from sinus attacks during change of season or on exposure to cold air.

Treatment

- Ceramic crescent-type magnets are applied on both sides of the nose for 10 minutes in the morning and 10 minutes in the evening.
- Drinking magnetised water four times helps in overcoming allergies, which lead to increased mucus production.
- Diseases like sneezing, coryza, allergic rhinitis and polypus can also be treated by application of magnets.
- The North Pole of ceramic magnet is applied on the right side of the nose while the South Pole is applied on the left side of the nose.

Constipation

- This is a disease of the large intestines, where the stools are hard, dry and evacuated with difficulty.
- The patient may have small and frequent stools also or incomplete expulsion with a sensation of stool remaining in the intestines and an unclear feeling.

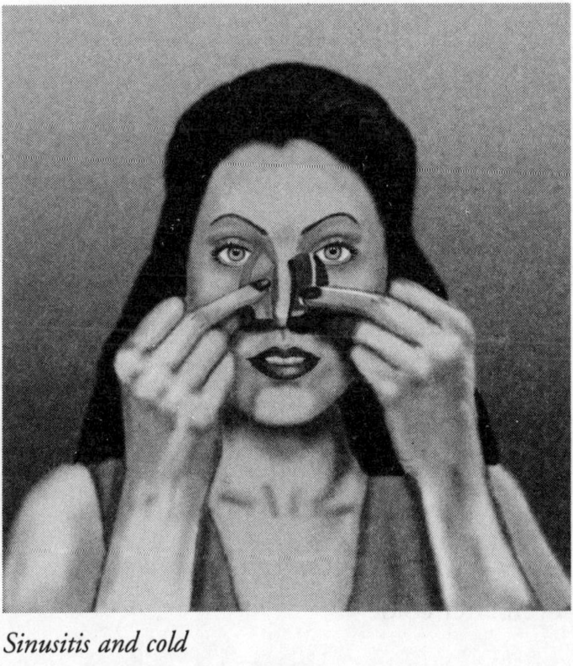

Sinusitis and cold

- It is caused by inadequate intake of water, no roughage in the diet, diseases like piles, intestinal obstruction, diverticulus— fissures, chronic amoebiasis and colitis, etc, sedentary habits, addictions to coffee, opium, drugs, etc, and certain allopathic drugs.

Treatment

- Drink plenty of water.
- Take ample amount of salads in the diet to make the roughage.
- Intake of dry figs and honey in warm water helps. Hot milk at bedtime also helps to regularise the bowel movements.
- Magnetic stomach belt is to be worn daily for at least 1 hour in the morning and evening.
- Drink magnetised water four times a day.

Tonsillitis

- These are glands situated in the throat.
- They get swollen or infected by the food we eat or even after cold.

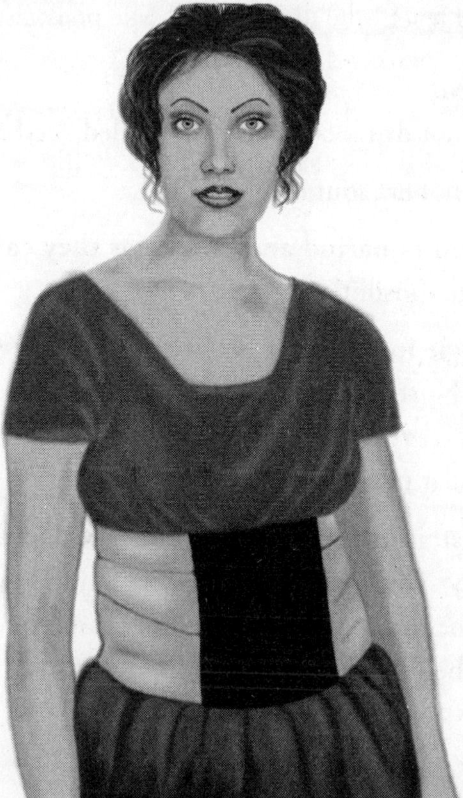

Abdominal ailments

- They may become septic at times and may lead to high fever.

Treatment

- Do not drink cold water or chilled, iced things.
- Do not eat sour or oily food.
- Avoid tamarind and pickles as they can cause acute tonsillitis.
- Gargle four times a day with magnetic water of the North pole, if the tonsils are septic. MWSP can treat chronic tonsillitis by gargling with bipolar magnetised water.
- Ceramic low power magnets can be applied twice daily. The North Pole is placed on the right side of the throat while the South Pole on the left side of the throat, for 10 to 15 minutes.